Keto With
The Ultimate Ketc

Eloise Richards

ELOISE RICHARDS

Keto Without Compromise

ELOISE RICHARDS

Contents:

Introduction

Comfort Food Cookbook

ELOISE RICHARDS

Keto Without Compromise
The Ultimate Keto Comfort Food Cookbook

INTRODUCTION

Dieting is always going to be important when you want to maintain a certain standard of living that doesn't compromise your health and wellness. Naturally, you only have one life to live. You always want to make the most out of it. You are going to want to indulge in as many guilty pleasures as you can. You will want to pursue the things that bring the most joy and happiness to your heart. However, you also have to balance it with mindfulness. You also have to make sure that you aren't compromising your physical self, and this is where dieting comes in.

Everyone knows that having a slice of pizza and a milkshake for every meal isn't exactly going to translate into good physical health. As delicious as these food items might be, they are often associated or linked to the declining health standards of people all over the world. According to an article by The Lancet, around one in five deaths are caused by poor dietary habits (Afshin 2017). One out of five might not seem like that big of a chunk, but if you look at it in terms of an actual figure, it translates into 11 million people. Now that is no number to laugh at. This study revealed that the deaths were primarily caused by a lack of consumption in whole grains, fruits, and vegetables in favor of processed meats, trans fats, and processed sugars. Based on a study by Statista, 31.3% of adults in the United States are classified as obese (2019). And obesity is widely known to be linked to many illnesses and health conditions such as heart disease and cancer.

Fortunately, more and more people are making a genuine effort to become conscious of what they eat and how much they consume. There is a whole new sub-industry that is emerging within the umbrella food industry as a whole that caters entirely to healthy eating. Of course, the fitness industry is booming with all sorts of training programs, personal coaching services, and diet regimens that are readily available for public consumption. However, for this book, we are going to focus on the latter: dieting.

Yes, it's true that diet regimens seem to be popping up everywhere lately. Every day, you probably encounter someone talking about a whole new diet program that they are on. You may have met someone on the Mediterranean diet or they're strictly following a Paleo diet. Some people like to talk about intermittent fasting, Atkins, South Beach, Zone, and all sorts of other diet fads out there. While these dietary programs do have their share of strengths as well, this book highlights one plan in particular: keto.

If you are familiar with mainstream media and pop culture, you probably know or have an idea of what the ketogenic diet is. A friend, gym companion, or someone's mother has more than likely approached you and told you about the benefits. You have probably seen the headlines of articles or covering it or watched a video on YouTube video of someone raving about keto. You might be thinking that there is nothing new in this book that you don't already know, but this isn't another book highlighting the same old information that you're familiar with. This is going to change your mind about keto.

We talked about how people need to find a balance between having fun and making the most out of life without ultimately compromising or destroying one's health. However, it's also essential that one doesn't always deprive oneself of life's great pleasures and indulgences. There must always be a balance. That is an idea that sets this book apart from other dietary guides or briefer. While this is a cookbook, it also focuses on keto recipes and meals that cater to a specific taste - an indulgent one.

See, you won't have to compromise eating your favorite foods just because you're on a diet. It's still very much possible for you to live a happy and healthy lifestyle while indulging in your go-to comfort food. This book highlights various recipes that focus on keeping your stomach full and your heart happy. Before we get to the recipes, you will be given a short explanation of the keto diet, its benefits, and how you can have fun with food even on a diet.

Life is composed primarily of one's pursuit of happiness. If you don't do things that make you happy, whether directly or indirectly, then what's the point of doing it? Sure, you might feel healthy if you munch on salads for every single meal. But would you be happy doing so? Looking at this book should prove as a valuable source of wellness and happiness for you. And hopefully, by the end, you will have gained a more profound understanding of the keto diet. You will know you don't have to skimp on delicious food for you to stay happy and fit.

What is Keto?

Before we jump right into the cooking, it's a good idea for you to gain a deeper, more profound understanding of what keto is and why this diet so popular today. After all, you never want to jump into a pool without knowing how deep it is first, right? You are always going to want to familiarize yourself with a diet program's philosophies before you try it out for yourself. Granted, if you already have a good grasp of what the keto diet is, feel free to skip on to other sections and get right into what benefits you the most. It's always good to refresh your memory on the core principles of the keto diet so that you can execute it properly. After all, you never know when you might learn something new. Don't be so quick to shut yourself off just yet.

So, what is keto? Well, keto in itself isn't a word. It has just gradually evolved to become the standard reference to the ketogenic diet. In a nutshell, the keto diet was designed to induce a state of ketosis in the body. But what exactly does ketosis mean? Ketosis is a metabolic state of the human body wherein there is an increased production of ketone bodies within one's metabolic system. Often a state of ketosis in the human body is only achieved when there is a drastic restriction in the consumption of carbohydrates. In simpler terms, the keto diet is essentially a diet that is geared to trigger ketosis by making sure that you aren't eating excessive carbs. Instead of focusing on the consumption of carbohydrates, proponents of the keto diet encourage a minimal intake of carbs, moderate consumption of protein, and a large consumption of fats.

Keto: A Brief Science Lesson

If you take the time to take a look at a diet's history, that is the best way to know if it's a fad or not. If a diet has been around for a long time and has a rich history, chances are it has proven its stripes as an effective weight loss solution. Before we get into the science behind the keto diet and why it can be a useful tool for weight loss and fitness regimen, a brief history lesson will do you some good.

It might be hard to believe, especially these days, that the roots of the ketogenic diet weren't founded initially on weight loss at all. People tend to turn towards the keto diet to trigger high metabolic function for the sole purpose of burning some extra fat. There are plenty of benefits to gain from fat loss. For one, a lot of people want to subscribe to a certain physical standard that is constantly being perpetuated by mainstream media. Somehow, they tell themselves that the leaner a person is, the more attractive they are going to be. However, it also cuts a lot deeper than that. There are plenty of people out there who want to lose weight for health reasons. Being fat and obese could potentially put one at risk of developing some very serious physical conditions like diabetes and heart disease. But everyone knows the struggles that are involved with shedding weight and burning fat. It's not an easy process and it can often take a lot of time and effort. Also, more than anything else, it's going to require a lot of dedication. Sometimes, that dedication has to take form of people having to give up certain culinary indulgences and guilty pleasures. And that's just not something that a lot of people are going to be willing to put themselves through. That's why the keto diet is practically a godsend for people who can't seem to give up their love and affinity for fatty food. For a lot of people all over the world, the keto diet is a method for them to lose weight while still eating their favorite food.

However, it wasn't always like that. Initially, people were made to fast and abstain from carb consumption to treat seizures and epileptic fits. The human body naturally functions off of glucose that comes from the carbohydrates you consume. At any given time, the human body stores around 2,000 calories' worth of glucose in the liver and your muscles. Normally, your body would be able to burn through all of those calories in the span of 48 hours. Once those calories have been used up, then the body needs to turn to alternative sources for fuel. This is when it automatically shifts into a ketogenic state. Instead of relying on stored glucose from carbohydrates, the body then proceeds to take stored fat and converts it into ketones. It was in the 1920s when a doctor from the Mayo Clinic called Russell Wilder, M.D. used this science as a way to combat epilepsy. He drew up dietary programs to be able to deplete the amount of sugar in the body to induce a ketogenic state. This treatment was shown to be a useful tool in fighting seizures and ever since keto principles have been used as a means to combat epileptic symptoms.

However, it never really stayed that way. It was in 1972 when Dr. Robert Atkins, M.D. first came out with his book talking about the Atkins diet. It was an instant hit, and it managed to gain some serious ground within a short amount of time. The first few weeks of his diet program had dieters eating copious amounts of fat while simultaneously limiting carbs as much as possible to stimulate weight loss. These were all the mechanics and ideas that were consistent with keto principles.

Little by little, more and more scientists, researchers, and even celebrities were jumping on the keto bandwagon. The keto diet has gradually evolved into becoming an amazing phenomenon as a result of its rich history. Every single day, more and more people are benefitting from adhering to keto principles. And it's not that hard to figure out that this is a diet program that is going to cement its place in the mainstream conversation for a very long time.

Pros of Being on a Keto Diet

Now that you have a better understanding of the keto diet and its origins, it's time to learn how you stand to benefit from the keto diet. You never want to jump on the bandwagon just because it's the thing to do, especially if it affects your health. You also want to make sure that you fully understand what it is you have to gain from a specific dietary principle. If you're still not convinced, then hopefully this section of the book you will help change your mind.

Helps You Lose Weight

Of course, the first and most popular benefit of adopting keto is that it's going to help you lose weight. Contrary to popular belief, eating lots of fat isn't necessarily going to make you fat. On a keto diet, you are encouraged to consume high amounts of fat instead of carbohydrates to induce a state of ketosis in the body. When the body is in a ketogenic state, it optimizes the body's metabolic rate. As a result, the human body ends up burning more excess fat even when the body is at rest. It's all about making sure that your metabolic rate is always functioning optimally. Fortunately, the keto diet is one that helps promote a healthy metabolism.

Helps Reduce the Effects of Acne

If you are a person who puts a lot of effort and care into your skincare routine, then it would be happy to know the keto diet helps reduce the effects of acne. Naturally, many factors play into a person's likelihood to develop acne. A lot of it has to do with genetics and a person's overall biological makeup. However, lifestyle plays a massive role in it as well. Blood sugar is linked to acne, and by eliminating carb intake, a person is more likely to be able to stave off acne.

Helps Reduce the Risk of Cancer

Unbeknownst to a lot of people, the ketogenic diet is utilized as a tool to prevent and even treat particular forms of cancer. A comprehensive study by Allen et. al found that the keto diet might also be a very potent supplementary treatment alongside radiation and chemotherapy (2014). The same studies concluded that this was because the keto diet would cause significant oxidative stress upon the cancer cells.

Aids in Brain Function

There is substantial research that needs to be conducted determining the ties between the keto diet and cognitive function. However, a study conducted by Halbook, Ji, Maudsley, and Martin found that kids who were strictly following the keto diet had better alertness and brain function (2011). Various research efforts are looking into the neuroprotective benefits of adopting the keto lifestyle.

Improves Cardiovascular Health

Ketogenic diets can also vastly aid in cardiovascular health. For the longest time, fat has always been tainted as the greatest enemy of the heart. You see a picture of bacon somewhere, and you also see a picture of a battered and torn up heart beside it. These are the kinds of ads that are always being shoved down peoples' throats. However, there is evidence that shows that the adoption of the ketogenic diet can improve cardiovascular health by reducing the body's cholesterol levels. A study found that HDL (or good cholesterol) levels also increased following the adoption of a keto diet (Dashti, 2004).

Improves Health of PCOS Patients

PCOS or polycystic ovarian syndrome is a condition that causes inflamed ovaries and cysts. This is an endocrine disorder that impacts women all over the world. High consumption of carbohydrates can contribute to the adverse effects and symptoms that are associated with PCOS. here aren't too many clinical studies or experiments that have been done on the ketogenic diet and PCOS connections. However, a 24-week study by Mavropolous, Yancy, Hepburn, and Westman found that the ketogenic diet helped fought off PCOS symptoms in five women (2005).

Reduces the Likelihood of Seizures

As previously mentioned, the origins of the keto diet are rooted in the combating of seizures and epileptic disorders. When a person is in a state of ketosis, they are less likely to experience seizures even when they are suffering from an epileptic condition.

Lowers the Risk of Diabetes

Diabetes is a deadly disease that is often closely associated with people who have large guts or a lot of fat in their midsection. Since the keto diet promotes effective weight loss and fat burn, it can also indirectly helps lower one's risk of contracting type 2 diabetes.

You Still Get to Have Fun With It

Let's face it. When you think of fun eating, your mind isn't always going to wander to salads, fruits, vegetables, or nuts. Fortunately, when you're on the keto diet, you don't have to give up your steaks, bacon, eggs, creams, cheeses, and other fatty foods. You might not be able to get your sugar fix the same way anymore. But at the very least, you still have the freedom to indulge in your favorite fatty foods. There is indeed an upside to going keto, but it might be a big turn off for people who are unwilling to give up some favorite foods.

This book exists to highlight the fact that you don't have to give up the comfort food that everyone craves from time to time. So next time you want to pick up that piece of fried chicken you won't have to think twice while on the keto diet. But more on that later.

Tips to Be Successful at Keto

Even though the keto lifestyle promotes the high consumption of fat, that doesn't mean that you should be eating all the cheese and oil you want. You can, but that's not how this diet works. You should always be making sure that you are doing keto the right way in order to achieve your goals. If you want to have success with keto, there are a few tips and principles that you are going to want to keep in mind throughout the entire process. Just because the keto diet paradigm is very broad doesn't mean that you won't have your share of responsibilities in practice. Here are a few tips that you might want to follow to make the most out of the keto experience:

Incorporate Intermittent Fasting into Your Routine

Sometimes, the best way to get the most out of a dietary program is to integrate another nutritional philosophy. There is a lot to gain from merging keto and intermittent fasting principles into one, especially if your goal is to lose weight. To engage in intermittent fasting means that you abstain from taking in any calories during a given amount of time. The most common template that people use for intermittent fasting is the 16:8 method. That means that you should only be consuming your food within an 8-hour window and that you should be fasting for the other 16 hours. Fasting and restricting yourself from consuming calories can aid in promoting ketosis in the body more efficiently.

Get Adequate Amounts of Sleep

The one aspect of a person's lifestyle that most individuals tend to forget when looking for success on a diet: sleep. Whenever you lack sleep, then there is a good chance that the stress hormones in your body are going to increase.

Whenever that happens, your ketogenic state ends up becoming compromised. It becomes more difficult for the human body to enter a state of ketosis when it's trying to fight off stress. At the very least, human adults should be getting around 7-9 hours of sleep on a nightly basis. If you have trouble sleeping at night, you can try lowering the temperature of your bedroom. That is known to help induce drowsiness. If that doesn't work, then you can also indulge in a natural sleeping aid such as melatonin.

Engage in Regular Exercise

If the goal here is to lose weight, then you're going to have to get active. Yes, going on a keto diet can help your body burn fat and lose weight more efficiently. it's still going to require a calorie count. You always want to make sure that you are using more calories than you are taking in. Even if you are on a ketogenic diet, if you are eating more calories than you're using up, you're still going to end up losing weight. Not to mention, engaging in a fit and active lifestyle can do wonders for your health and wellness.

Refrain from Drinking Soda Substitutes

Just because soda substitutes claim to have "zero sugar" doesn't mean that it's free reign to over-indulge while you're on a keto diet. These drinks with sugar alternatives or substitutes indeed have zero carbohydrates. However, these substitutes contain chemicals that trick the human body into thinking that you're consuming sugar. When that happens, it makes it harder for your body to enter a ketogenic state. Artificial sweeteners should still be considered as carbohydrates even with have zero calories.

Stay Hydrated

Regardless of your diet, it's essential to always stay hydrated. Remember that 73% of the human body is comprised of water. You have to take note of the fact that your body is losing a lot more water when you're not taking in enough carbohydrates. You can be at risk of dehydrating yourself on the keto diet if you aren't actively tracking the amount of water that you are drinking. And to be safe, if you live in a warmer climate you are primarily going to want to make sure that you are drinking more than the average amount of water.

Get Your Carbs from Leafy Vegetables

Just because you shouldn't eat too many carbohydrates doesn't mean that you are free from eating your veggies. You always stand to benefit from eating green leafy vegetables. The great thing about these green vegetables is that they usually tend to have very low caloric compositions while still being loaded with a lot of valuable vitamins and minerals. These vegetables are also going to serve as great sources of fiber, which can help maintain a healthy bowel. Examples of these vegetables include kale, spinach, lettuce, cauliflower, cabbage, and Brussels sprouts.

Count Your Macros

Okay. You are still going to have to do a little math while you're on the keto diet whether you like it or not. But you don't have to worry. This isn't going to be any complicated trigonometry or calculus. You have to make sure that you are keeping track of your macros. What are macros? Macros or macronutrients are the three major nutrients, namely: carbohydrates, protein, and fats. You want to make sure that you are actively tracking the numbers behind your macros so that you can better police your food consumption. If you don't count your macros, you are at risk of eating too many carbohydrates which prevents you from entering a ketogenic state.

Make Use of Coconut Oil

Don't just rub it onto your skin. That may feel nice but it won't help achieve a ketogenic state. Incorporate coconut oil into your diet because by ingesting this nutrient rich oil it makes it easier for your body to achieve ketosis. Coconut oil is packed with medium-chain triglycerides or MCTs. MCT is a special kind of fat that is more efficiently absorbed by the liver where ketones are produced. Coconut oil is one of the most effective things you can eat to induce ketosis in your body.

Having Fun with Keto

It's a lot easier to stick to doing something when you're having fun in the process. That's why it's always important that you can incorporate a little bit of fun into all of the things that you do in life. This is especially true when you are on a diet. It can be very easy to get discouraged while on a diet when you always feel miserable or sad about your situation. Like if you are always feeling sorry for yourself because you can't eat what you want. You are more likely to abandon or dropping your diet altogether because of the unhappiness it is causing you.

However, if you are making a genuine effort to have fun on your diet, then it becomes a lot easier to stay committed to it. It won't have to feel like a chore, job, or responsibility. That is exactly what this book is going to try to help. As already mentioned in this book, you don't have to compromise fun when you are on the keto diet. You are still encouraged to eat the food that brings happiness to your soul so as long as this food doesn't keep you from achieving ketosis.

This is where creativity steps in. Sometimes, you're just going to have to think outside of the box by coming up with food hacks to make your dietary experience a more enjoyable one. You might think it will be easy to eat large quantities of fatty food. It will be at the beginning, but over time, it will become challenging to find your appetite if you're eating the same thing over and over again. You always want to try mixing things up every once in a while.

Comfort food is always going to play a very prominent role in anyone's culinary experience. By its name, comfort food is designed to bring a sense of ease and peace to one's soul. While on the keto diet, you don't have to give up your precious comfort food. As you embark on this dietary journey, you should know that you don't have to limit yourself too much, if at all. There is still a way for you to enjoy all of your favorite food without compromising your dietary goals. With the help of this book, you can make this happen.

Before you move on from this introduction, you must know that you don't necessarily have to follow the recipes in this cookbook exactly. Feel free to get creative and add your spin to things because you're going to eat this food anyway. It's important to enjoy the whole process so that you won't ever feel discouraged.

Comfort Food Cookbook

Chapter 1: Breakfast

Keto Pancakes

Servings: 3

Prep Time: 5 minutes

Cook Time: 10 minutes

Calories per serving: 244 kcal

Macros:

- Fat: 23 g

- Protein: 5.5 g

- Carbs: 5 g

Ingredients:

- ½ cup of coconut flour

- ½ tsp of baking soda

- 2 tbsp of melted coconut oil

- 1 tsp of vanilla

- 4 \ medium-sized organic eggs

- ½ tsp of cinnamon

- ½ cup of coconut cream

- ½ cup of unsweetened almond milk

- ¼ tsp of sea salt

Instructions:

1. Add all of the ingredients into a high-powered blender.

2. Blend all of the ingredients until you achieve a nice and smooth consistency throughout.

3. Take a medium-sized skillet and heat it over medium heat.

4. Add non-stick oil or butter to the pan (optional).

5. When the pan is heated, pour approximately ½ of a cup of the mixed batter into the skillet.

6. Cook the batter until the surface starts to bubble and it is golden on the underside.

7. Flip and cook the other side until it achieves the same golden color.

8. Repeat the process until the batter runs out.

9. Feel free to add your favorite keto-friendly toppings like berries, peanut butter, or cream.

Keto French Toast

Servings: 2

Prep Time: 5 minutes

Cook Time: 15 minutes

Calories per serving: 683 kcal

Macros:

- Fat: 58 g

- Protein: 29 g

- Carbs: 17 g

-

Ingredients:

- 1 loaf of paleo bread (either coconut flour or almond flour is permissible)

- 1 tbsp of butter

- ⅓ cup of coconut yogurt

- 2 tsp of stevia

- 1 tsp of vanilla extract

- garnishes to serve: berries, cacao nibs, shredded coconut, etc. (optional)

Instructions:

1. Take your paleo bread loaf and slice it into three pieces. After that, take each slice and cut it in half lengthwise to make six different pieces of bread.

2. Take a large frying pan and heat the butter on medium heat. Swirl the butter all over the pan.

3. When the pan is heated, take two slices of bread and cook on each side until a golden

brown color and toasted consistency is achieved.

4. While waiting for the bread to toast, prepare a medium bowl for the yogurt topping mixture.

5. Add coconut yogurt, stevia, and vanilla into the bowl. Whisk or whip the yogurt mixture until it begins to thicken. Add more stevia or vanilla to the mixture according to taste.

6. Take the toasted bread slices and place it on a plate. Top with yogurt mixture and selected garnishes.

McDonald's-Inspired Keto Sausage Egg McMuffin

Servings: 1

Prep Time: 10 minutes

Cook Time: 10 minutes

Calories per serving: 687 kcal

Macros:

- Fat: 61 g

- Protein: 32 g

- Carbs: 4 g

Ingredients:

- 2 tbsp of butter

- ¼ lb of raw pork breakfast sausage

- 2 large eggs

- ¼ cup of water

- 2 tbsp of guacamole (optional)

- salt and pepper to taste

Instructions:

1. Take two stainless steel biscuit cutters that are around 3 and ½ inches in size. Grease the insides of the cutters with melted butter. Place one cutter on a plate and insert the sausage meat inside of it.

2. Gently press down on the meat to make sure that the patty is neatly shaped and uniform.

3. Take a skillet and put it over medium heat. Add a tablespoon of butter and allow to

heat for a bit. Once the butter is shimmering, add the sausage patty into the pan. If you wish to preserve the integrity of the shape of the patty, you can leave the biscuit cutters on until the patty has shrunk.

4. Take the biscuit cutter from the pan and repeat the greasing process with melted butter.

5. Fry the sausage in the pan for around 2 or 3 minutes on each side. If the patty is thick, then you might want to cover the pan to make sure that it's cooked through. Once the sausage patty is cooked, transfer it onto a plate.

6. To make the keto buns, you are going to have to crack two eggs into two separate

bowls. Pierce the yolk of the egg with a fork.

7. Take a skillet and place it over medium-high heat. Add a tablespoon of butter to the skillet. Take two biscuit cutters that have already been greased and place it on top of the skillet. Pour an egg into each cutter.

8. Season the eggs with salt and pepper to taste.

9. Slowly add ¼ cup of water to the skillet outside of the egg molds.

10. Turn the heat down to low and cover the pan with a tight-fitting lid. Cook the eggs

all the way through. This should take around 3 minutes.

11. Once cooked, transfer the eggs onto a plate that's lined with a paper towel.

12. Use the eggs as the "bread" for the "Mc-Muffin" sandwich. Add some guacamole for added flavor and texture within the sandwich. For a little extra kick, feel free to put some sriracha too.

Chocolate "Ketoatmeal"

Servings: 2

Prep Time: 5 minutes

Cook Time: 10 minutes

Calories per serving: 450 kcal

Macros:

- Fat: 42 g

- Protein: 24 g

- Carbs: 18 g

Ingredients:

- 1 medium sized cauliflower head (steamed and riced)

- 1 tablespoon coconut oil

- 1 cup coconut milk

- 4 large eggs (beaten)

- 1 and ½ tbsp of cacao powder

- 1 scoop of collagen protein powder

- ¼ tsp of salt

- 1 scoop of Mitosweet

- 1 tbsp of stevia

- cacao nibs, berries, or shredded coconut to garnish (optional)

Instructions:

1. When you are using a whole cauliflower for this recipe, make sure that you chop it into little florets first.

2. Take the florets and place it into a blender or food processor until it achieves a rice-

like consistency. This is your cauliflower rice.

3. Take a wide saucepan and add the coconut milk. Bring it to a light simmer.

4. Add the cauliflower rice to the coconut milk and stir. Bring the heat down to low and allow the cauliflower to thicken. This process should take roughly around 4 minutes.

5. Take the beaten eggs and add into the pan gently.

6. Add cacao powder, protein powder, Mito-Sweet, salt, and stevia into the pan.

7. Stir the mixture gently and allow the eggs to cook thoroughly. Once eggs are cooked and the cauliflower has thickened even further, stir the mixture again.

8. Top with selected garnishes and serve.

Keto Fried Rice

Servings: 3

Prep Time: 10 minutes

Cook Time: 10 minutes

Calories per serving: 327 kcal

Macros:

- Fat: 25 g

- Protein: 12 g

- Carbs:13 g

Ingredients:

- 4 slices of bacon

- 2 tbsp of olive oil

- 8 oz of cauliflower (steamed and riced)

- 1 small diced onion

- 1 small diced red bell pepper

- 6 oz of broccoli florets

- 2 tsp of coconut aminos

- 3 large eggs

- salt and pepper to taste

- sliced green onion for garnish

Instructions:

1. When you are using a whole cauliflower for this recipe, make sure that you chop it into little florets first.

2. Take the florets and place it into a blender or food processor until it achieves a rice-like consistency. This is your cauliflower rice. Set the rice aside for a moment.

3. Take a medium-sized skillet and place it over medium-high heat. Once the skillet is hot, add bacon and bring to a sizzle. Cook bacon until crisp and browned on all sides. Once the bacon is cooked, remove it from the skillet and place it on a plate.

4. Leave the bacon fat in the skillet and add 2 tablespoons of olive oil there for some extra fat.

5. Bring the heat down to medium and add the onions to the skillet.

6. Cook the onions until they are soft and translucent. Season the onions with salt and pepper, and continue to cook even further.

7. Add the broccoli to the skillet and cook it with the fat and onions. Season it with more salt and pepper. Cover the skillet for about 30-45 seconds to allow the broccoli to cook and soften.

8. Take the lid off the skillet and add the cauliflower rice, chopped bacon, and coconut aminos into the skillet. Stir the ingredients to make sure that the cauliflower rice is properly coated by the bacon and broccoli. Continue to cook until the cauliflower rice completely softens.

9. Bring the heat down to low.

10. In a separate skillet, cook eggs to your own preference. Once your eggs are

cooked, add to a plate together with the cauliflower fried rice.

11. Garnish with thinly sliced green onions.

Chapter 2: Lunch

Pepperoni Pizza Meatloaf

Servings: 10

Prep Time: 10 minutes

Cook Time: 40 minutes

Calories per serving: 350 kcal

Macros:

- Fat: 19 g

- Protein: 41 g

- Carbs: 2 g

Ingredients:

- 3 lbs of ground turkey meat

- 2 medium-sized eggs

- 1 tbsp of garlic powder

- 1 tbsp of onion powder

- 1 tbsp of minced garlic

- 1 tbsp of minced onion

- 2 tsp of oregano

- 2 tsp of basil

- 2 tsp of parsley

- 16 oz of mozzarella cheese

- 5 oz of pepperoni

- salt and pepper to taste

- low-carb tomato sauce to serve

Instructions:

1. Preheat oven to 350 degrees F or 177 degrees C.

2. Cut the mozzarella cheese in half lengthwise into two pieces measuring 2 x 2 x 6 inches.

3. Take the ground turkey and place it into a large bowl. Combine the meat with eggs and spices.

4. Place ⅓ of the seasoned meat onto a baking pan forming a 7 x 10-inch rectangle.

5. Put a layer of pepperoni right in the middle of the meat.

6. Cover the sides and top of the meat with mozzarella and pepperoni.

7. Take the rest of the ground turkey and en-case the mozzarella and pepperoni.

8. Place the remaining pepperoni outside of the meatloaf.

9. Bake for around 40-50 minutes.

Keto Philly Cheesesteak Stuffed Peppers with Cauliflower

Servings: 6

Prep Time: 10 minutes

Cook Time: 50 minutes

Calories per serving: 379 kcal

Macros:

- Fat: 22.9 g

- Protein: 32.7 g

- Carbs: 11 g

Ingredients:

- 2 tbsp of olive oil

- 2 large onions, sliced

- 6 small halved and seeded green bell peppers

- 1 lb of very thinly sliced beef top sirloin steak

- 2 cups of sliced cauliflower

- 12 oz. of sliced Provolone cheese

- Salt to taste

Instructions:

1. Add olive oil onto a large pan over medium heat.

2. Add the onions into the pan and allow to sweat. Add just a dash of salt to season the onions.

3. Cook the onions until they are caramelized or if they have begun to change into a golden brown color.

4. Be careful not to burn the onions. Turn down the heat if you feel like the pan is getting a little too hot.

5. If done correctly, the onion cooking process should take around 30-40 minutes long.

6. While the onions are cooking, take the peppers and place them into a large pot with water in it and cover. Bring the water to a boil and allow to cook the peppers for around 2-3 minutes or until they start to soften up.

7. Drain the peppers and place them on a layer of paper towel. Pat the peppers dry until all moisture is eliminated.

8. Place the peppers into a 9 x 13-inch pan and preheat the oven to 350 degrees F or 177 degrees C.

9. Take a new pan and heat 1 tbsp of olive oil over medium heat. Once the pan is hot, cook the steak until it achieves a golden brown color and transfer to a plate once it has been cooked.

10. Take the beef and caramelized onions and season with sea salt. Mix the beef and caramelized onions together.

11. Stuff the bell peppers with the onion and beef mixture. Top off every pepper with a single slice of cheese. Place the peppers into the oven and allow to bake for around 10-15 minutes or until the cheese starts to melt.

12. Change the oven setting to a high broil and cook for around 2-4 minutes or until the cheese changes into a slightly golden brown.

13. Remove from oven and let rest for 2 minutes. Serve while hot.

Stir Fry Keto Zoodles

Servings: 4

Prep Time: 10 minutes

Cook Time: 10 minutes

Calories per serving: 150 kcal

Macros:

- Fat: 8 g

- Protein: 4 g

- Carbs: 13 g

Ingredients:

- 4 small spiraled or stringed zucchinis

- 2 spiraled or stringed yellow onions

- 2 tbsp of olive oil

- 1 tbsp of low sodium soy sauce

- 2 tbsp of teriyaki sauce

- 1 tbsp of sesame seeds

Instructions:

1. Pat the stringed or spiraled zucchinis with a paper towel to get rid of all the moisture.

2. Heat oil in a wok over medium heat.

3. Once the wok is heated, add the onions and allow to sweat for around 4 to 5 minutes.

4. Add the stringed zucchini into the wok and cook for another 2 minutes.

5. Add sauces and sesame seeds into the wok and cook for an extra 5 minutes or until zucchini is tender.

6. Add chopped red peppers for an extra kick (optional).

Ground Beef Casserole

Servings: 8

Prep Time: 10 minutes

Cook Time: 20 minutes

Calories per serving: 265 kcal

Macros:

- Fat: 15 g

- Protein: 28 g

- Carbs: 2 g

Ingredients:

- olive oil or non-stick spray

- 2 lbs of lean ground beef

- 1 tsp of sea salt

- ¼ tsp of black pepper

- 2 tsp of garlic powder

- 1 tsp of onion powder

- ¼ tsp of cayenne pepper

- 1 cup of shredded cheddar

- 4 oz of cubed reduced fat cream cheese

- 2 tbsp of chopped parsley

Instructions:

1. Preheat the oven to 400 degrees F or 204 degrees C. Spray 2-quart casserole dish with non-stick spray or olive oil and set aside.

2. Heat a large nonstick pan over medium-high heat. Coat with non-stick spray or olive oil.

3. Add the ground beef to the skillet and cook until meat is brown and cooked through. This should take around 5 minutes. Continuously sift and stir through the beef to make sure that it is all cooked through.

4. Reduce the heat of the stove to medium. Mix the pepper, salt, garlic powder, cayenne pepper, and onion powder into the beef to add more flavor and seasoning.

5. Add the cream cheese into the pan and mix thoroughly.

6. Turn the heat off and add ½ cup of shredded cheddar into the beef.

7. Transfer the contents of the pan into the casserole dish that you set aside earlier.

8. Sprinkle what is left of the shredded cheddar cheese on top of the casserole.

9. Bake the ground beef casserole for around 10 minutes or until the cheese starts to melt.

10. Add parsley for garnish and serve.

Keto Meatballs with Creamy Tomato Sauce

Servings: 8

Prep Time: 10 minutes

Cook Time: 30 minutes

Calories per serving: 414 kcal

Macros:

- Fat: 32 g

- Protein: 23 g

- Carbs: 12 g

Ingredients:

For the meatballs:

- 1 lb of lean ground pork

- 1 lb of lean ground chicken

- 2 cups of chopped spinach

- 2 cups of shredded zucchini

- 2 cloves of minced garlic

- 1 and ½ tsp of Italian seasoning

- 1 tsp of salt

- coconut oil for frying

For the tomato sauce:

- 2 tsp of coconut oil

- 4 cloves of garlic

- 2 14 oz cans of crushed tomatoes

- 1 cup of coconut cream

- 2 tsp of Italian seasoning

- 1 tsp of salt

- chopped parsley for garnish

Instructions:

1. Take all of the meatball ingredients and combine into a large mixing bowl. Mix all of the ingredients thoroughly until an acceptable consistency is achieved.

2. Portion the meatball mixture into equal-sized balls until all of the mixture has been used up.

3. Take a large skillet over medium heat and add coconut oil. Fry all of the meatballs until all of them are browned on all sides and cooked through. Transfer the meatballs to a plate once they are cooked.

4. In another skillet, heat up 2 tsp of coconut oil over medium-low heat.

5. Add the garlic into the skillet and allow to cook until fragrant. This should take approximately 30 seconds.

6. Add the remaining sauce ingredients and stir thoroughly.

7. Bring the entire sauce mixture to a low boil and then reduce the heat slightly. Allow to simmer for around 5-10 minutes. Return meatballs to the skillet and simmer for around 3-5 minutes.

8. Serve the meatballs and sauce over zucchini noodles and garnish with parsley.

Chapter 3: Dinner

Cauliflower Mac and Cheese

Servings: 4

Prep Time: 5 minutes

Cook Time: 20 minutes

Calories per serving: 294 kcal

Macros:

- Fat: 23 g

- Protein: 11 g

- Carbs: 12 g

Ingredients:

- 1 full head of cauliflower, cut and sliced into small florets

- 3 tbsp of butter

- 1 cup of shredded cheddar cheese

- ¼ cup of cream

- ¼ cup of unsweetened almond milk

- salt and pepper to taste

Instructions:

1. Preheat oven to 450 degrees F or 232 degrees C and line a baking sheet with parchment paper.

2. Melt 2 tbsp of butter.

3. Take cauliflower florets and pour into bowl with melted butter, salt, and pepper.

4. Place the cauliflower on the parchment paper on top of the baking sheet and roast for around 15 minutes or until crisp.

5. Pour shredded cheese, milk, and cream into a broiler and heat on top of the stove on medium-high heat. You can also opt to use a microwave for this.

6. Heat the mixture until it is smooth and bubbly. Be careful not to overcook the cheese to the point that it is burnt.

7. Toss cauliflower into the cheese mixture and serve.

Sausage and Cabbage Soup

Servings: 10

Prep Time: 10 minutes

Cook Time: 30 minutes

Calories per serving: 131 kcal

Macros:

- Fat: 21.3 g

- Protein: 17 g

- Carbs: 7 g

Ingredients:

- 1 lb of cooked and sliced Italian sausage

- 1 chopped onion

- 2 cloves of garlic, minced

- 7 cups of chopped cabbage

- 54 oz. of canned dried tomatoes

- 1 cup of water

- 2 tsp of basil

- 1 tsp of oregano

- ¼ tsp of rosemary

- 1 bay leaf

- ½ tsp of salt

- ¼ tsp of pepper

- 2 tsp of brown sugar

Instructions:

1. In a large pot, stir in all ingredients together and bring to a boil.

2. Cover and reduce heat to medium-low and simmer for 30 minutes to 1 hour.

3. Remove bay leaf and serve while hot.

Cheesy Broccoli Soup

Servings: 8

Prep Time: 5 minutes

Cook Time: 20 minutes

Calories per serving:

Macros:

- Fat: 25 g

- Protein: 13 g

- Carbs: 5 g

Ingredients:

- 4 cups of broccoli chopped into florets

- 4 cloves of minced garlic

- 3 and ½ cups of chicken broth

- 1 cup of full cream

- 3 cups of shredded cheddar cheese

Instructions:

1. Add oil or butter to a large pot over medium heat.

2. Once the pot is hot, add the chicken broth, cream, and chopped broccoli.

3. Increase the heat of the stove and bring the mixture to a boil.

4. Reduce heat and allow to simmer for 10-20 minutes or until the broccoli is tender and soft.

5. Gradually add the cheese into the simmering pot little by little continuously stirring the mixture throughout the entire process.

6. Keep on adding cheese until you run out completely. Never stop stirring.

7. Serve while hot.

Creamy Sundried Tomato and Parmesan Chicken Zucchini Noodles

Servings: 6

Prep Time: 15 minutes

Cook Time: 15 minutes

Calories per serving: 394 kcal

Macros:

- Fat: 22.6 g

- Protein: 35.6 g

- Carbs: 9.2 g

Ingredients:

- 1 tbsp of butter

- 1.5 lbs of skinless chicken thigh fillets, cut into strips

- 4 oz of chopped fresh semi-dried tomato strips in oil

- 3.5 oz of chopped jarred sun dried tomatoes in oil

- 4 cloves of garlic, peeled and crushed

- 1 ¼ cup of reduced fat or full fat thickened cream (or half and half)

- 1 cup of shaved Parmesan cheese

- Salt to taste

- Dried basil seasoning

- Red chili flakes

- 2 large Zucchinis made into zoodles (use a vegetable grater or zoodle grater)

Instructions:

1. Place butter or oil into a pan over medium high heat.

2. Add the chicken strips into the pan and generously season with salt.

3. Fry the chicken until it achieves a golden brown color on all sides. Make sure that the chicken is cooked through.

4. Add the tomatoes into the pan along with 1 tablespoon of oil. Add garlic and saute along with everything else to add some extra flavor.

5. While waiting for your chicken to cook, prepare your zoodles by stringing your zucchinis or by putting them through a zoodle maker or vegetable peeler.

6. Lower the heat of the pan, and add the cream along with the Parmesan cheese.

7. Allow the cheese to simmer while stirring continuously until the cheese has achieved a smooth melted consistency.

8. Season the contents of the pan with salt, basil, and chilli flakes to taste.

9. Add the zoodles and cook for around 5-8 minutes or until it's begun to soften.

Keto Chicken Pot Pie

Servings: 8

Prep Time: 3 hrs and 30 minutes

Cook Time: 22 minutes

Calories per serving: 300 kcal

Macros:

- Fat: 17 g

- Protein: 12 g

- Carbs: 6 g

Ingredients:

For the filling:

- ½ cup of mixed vegetables

- 2 and ½ cups of cooked chicken, diced

- ¼ tsp of Xanthan gum

- ¼ diced small onion

- 2 minced garlic cloves

- ¾ cup of full whipping cream

- 1 cup of chicken broth

- ¼ tsp of rosemary

- 1 tsp of poultry seasoning

- pinch of thyme

- 2 tbsp of butter

- salt and pepper to taste

For the crust:

- ⅓ cup of coconut flour

- 2 tbsp of full fat sour cream

- 4 medium-sized eggs

- ¼ tsp of baking powder

- 1 cup of mild grated cheese

- ⅓ cup of mozzarella cheese

- 4 and ½ tsp of melted butter

- 1 and ½ tsp of parsley for garnish

- ¼ tsp of salt

Instructions:

1. If chicken is still uncooked, then place into a slow cooker for around 3 hours on high heat or 6 hours on low heat.

2. Preheat the oven at 400 degrees F or 204 C.

3. Saute the onion, garlic cloves, and mixed vegetables in 2 tbsp of butter in an oven-

safe skillet. Season with salt and pepper. Cook until the onions are translucent.

4. Add the full whipping cream into the skillet along with thyme, rosemary, poultry seasoning, and chicken broth.

5. Sprinkle the Xantham gum on top and allow to simmer until the sauce achieves a thicker consistency. Make sure that while you simmer, you are covering the skillet to prevent the liquid from evaporating. Liquid is necessary in this recipe.

6. Add the cooked diced chicken into the skillet.

7. To make the breading, combine the melted butter with eggs, salt, and sour cream into a large bowl. Mix the ingredients thoroughly.

8. Add coconut flour and baking soda to the bowl and mix it thoroughly.

9. Stir in the cheese.

10. Drop the batter gradually by dollops into the chicken pot pie. Make sure that you don't spread it out too much as the coconut flour might absorb the liquid.

11. Bake in the oven for around 15 to 20 minutes.

12. Set the oven to broil and allow to broil for 1-2 minutes until the crust is crisp. Sprinkle the parsley on top as garnish.

Chapter 4: Snacks

Cheesy Keto Tater Tots

Servings: 6

Prep Time: 5 minutes

Cook Time: 15 minutes

Calories per serving: 145 kcal

Macros:

- Fat: 11 g

- Protein: 7 g

- Carbs: 4 g

Ingredients:

- 1 and ½ lbs of riced cauliflower (approx. 1 head)

- ¼ cup of olive oil

- 1 large egg

- 1 and ½ cup of mozzarella cheese

- 2 cloves of garlic

- ¾ tsp of salt

Instructions:

1. Stir fry the cauliflower rice with around 2 tbsp of olive oil in a large wok over medium-high heat. Cook until soft and lightly browned with no moisture left in the wok.

2. Whisk the egg in a large bowl. Add mozzarella, garlic, and salt.

3. Mix the egg and cheese mixture into the large wok along with the cauliflower rice while it's still hot. The heat should be able

to melt the cheese and make the mixture slightly sticky in consistency.

4. Take the mixture and form into 6 different tater tots or patties. Flatten them slightly to make sure that they are easier to cook all the way through.

5. Take a wide pan and heat 2 tbsp of olive oil over medium-high heat. Add the tater tots or patties in a single layer. Make sure that the tots don't come into contact with one another while cooking. Fry the tots for around 2 minutes on one side or until it's golden brown, and then flip for another 2 minutes of cooking on the other side.

6. Repeat this cooking process until all of the tater tots are cooked.

Keto Pretzel Bites

Servings: 8

Prep Time: 15 minutes

Cook Time: 15 minutes

Calories per serving: 315 kcal

Macros:

- Fat: 24 g

- Protein: 18 g

- Carbs:8 g

Ingredients:

- 3 cups of skim low moisture shredded mozzarella cheese

- 2 oz of cream cheese

- 3 medium-sized eggs

- 2 cups of almond flour

- 1 tbsp of baking powder

- 1 tbsp of salt

Instructions:

1. Preheat the oven to 400 degrees F or 204 degrees C.

2. Line a baking sheet with a baking mat or parchment paper.

3. In a medium-sized bowl, mix together the baking powder and almond flour. Whisk thoroughly and set aside.

4. In a large microwavable bowl, add the cream cheese and mozzarella. Make sure

that the cream cheese is at the bottom of the bowl and the mozzarella is on top so that the latter gets most exposure to the microwave.

5. Melt the cheese inside the microwave for 30 seconds at full power. Take the bowl out of the microwave and stir. Place the bowl back into the microwave and repeat this process until the cheese is completely melted all the way through. Make sure that you don't overdo it by burning the cheese.

6. All in all, the microwaving process should take roughly around 2 minutes or so. It's important that you don't microwave the cheese all at once or else it will end up burning.

7. Once the cheese has melted, add it along with the flour mixture and 2 eggs into a food processor. Pulse at a high speed until the dough has achieved an acceptable consistency. The dough might end up really sticky, but that is only to be expected.

8. Wrap your pastry board with a plastic wrap and make sure the wrap is taut. Make sure that the wrap is rolled all the way through to the bottom of the board so that it doesn't move around while you go on with your preparations. The plastic wrap is there to prevent your dough from sticking to the pastry board.

9. Divide the dough into roughly around 8 equal parts and roll them into ropes that are around 1 inch thick.

10. Take a knife and slice the dough into ¾ inch pieces. This should amount to roughly around 72-75 bites overall. Place the bites onto the baking sheet that you prepared earlier.

11. Take the last egg and put it into a bowl. Whisk the egg. This will serve as the wash. Brush the surfaces of the pretzels with egg wash. Season the tops of the pretzels with salt.

12. Bake the pretzels for around 12 minutes or until they have turned into a light golden brown color. After that, set the oven to broil and cook for another 2 minutes. This will allow for a crisping to take place on the exteriors of the pretzel. It's important that during these final two minutes, you pay at-

tention to your pretzels to prevent them from burning.

13. Remove from oven and allow to cool.

Keto Egg Drop Soup

Servings: 2

Prep Time: 2 minutes

Cook Time: 5 minutes

Calories per serving: 88 kcal

Macros:

- Fat: 6 g

- Protein: 8 g

- Carbs: 1 g

Ingredients:

- 200 ml of bone broth

- 2 eggs

- parsley for garnish

Instructions:

1. Place the bone broth into a large pot and bring it to a boil.

2. While waiting for the broth to boil, take a separate bowl and mix in the two eggs with a fork.

3. Once the broth has been brought to a simmer, gradually add the egg mixture into the broth. Keep stirring throughout the entire process.

4. Serve in a bowl and add parsley for garnish.

Crispy Brussels Sprouts and Bacon

Servings: 4

Prep Time: 5 minutes

Cook Time: 20 minutes

Calories per serving: 240 kcal

Macros:

- Fat: 19 g

- Protein: 6 g

- Carbs: 11 g

Ingredients:

- 4 slices of bacon

- 1 lb of halved brussels sprouts

- 3 tbsp of extra virgin olive oil

- ¾ tsp of salt

- ¼ tsp of black pepper

- 2 tbsp of balsamic vinegar

Instructions:

1. Place a large saute pan on the stove and turn the heat to medium. Add the bacon into the pan and fry the slices until both sides are crispy.

2. Remove the bacon and set aside. Allow the bacon to drain on dry paper towels. Do not remove the bacon grease that is within the pan.

3. Add 2 tbsp of olive oil to the pan and allow to swirl around. Add the brussels sprouts

into the pan and allow to cook. Season with salt and black pepper.

4. Increase the heat of the pan to a medium-high. Arrange the brussels sprouts in a single layer. Sear the sprouts for around 4 minutes or until it is thoroughly browned on the bottom. Flip the sprouts and repeat the browning process on the other side.

5. While waiting for the sprouts to cook, chop the bacon slices.

6. Add balsamic vinegar and 1 tbsp of olive oil into the pan along with the brussels sprouts and allow to cook for another 2 minutes.

7. Return the bacon to the pan and mix it all together.

Zucchini Boats with Buffalo Chicken

Servings: 4

Prep Time: 15 minutes

Cook Time: 40 minutes

Calories per serving: 408 kcal

Macros:

- Fat: 21 g

- Protein: 21 g

- Carbs: 3 g

Ingredients:

- 4 medium-sized zucchinis

- 2 tbsp of olive oil

- 3 cups of cooked chicken breast, shredded

- 1 cup plain greek yogurt

- 3 minced garlic cloves

- ¼ diced red onion

- ⅓ cup of Tabasco

- 1 and ¼ cup of shredded cheddar cheese

- ¼ cup of ranch dressing

- thinly sliced scallions for garnish

Instructions:

1. Preheat the oven to 400 degrees F or 204 degrees C. Grease a large baking pan with oil and set to the side for a while.

2. Take the zucchinis and slice them in half lengthwise. Ideally, your zucchinis would be similar in size.

3. Take a spoon and hollow out the insides of the zucchini. Leave about ½ inch rim for you to create the boat. Place the hollowed zucchinis onto the baking pan and set aside for a while.

4. Add 1 tablespoon of olive oil onto a medium skillet and place it over medium heat. Once the skillet is hot, add onions and garlic. Saute for around 3 to 4 minutes or until the onions become soft and translucent. Once cooked, transfer the contents of the skillet into a large bowl.

5. Add the cooked chicken, hot sauce, greek yogurt, ranch dressing, hot sauce, and shredded cheddar cheese into the bowl. Mix the contents of the bowl thoroughly. This will serve as the buffalo chicken stuffing for the zucchini boats.

6. Take a spoon and gradually transfer the buffalo chicken stuffing into the hollowed out zucchinis. Top each boat with the remaining amount of cheddar cheese.

7. Cover all of the zucchini boats with foil and bake for around 40-45 minutes or until the zucchini has softened and the cheese has melted. Once the zucchini has turned tender, remove the foil from the tops of the boats. Set the oven to broil and allow the boats to broil for around 2-3 minutes. This

process will help brown and crisp the cheese slightly.

8. Once done baking, take the boats out of the oven and allow to cool. Garnish with green onions.

Conclusion

The keto journey might not necessarily be one that all people are going to want to take. But hopefully, this book was able to provide you with a unique perspective and insight into what the keto diet is truly all about. At the end of the day, food is always going to play a very important aspect of a person's life. There is a reason why the food industry is worth trillions of dollars worldwide. It's something that every single one of us relates to as food is very near and dear to our hearts.

For the more pragmatic, food is seen as a source of nourishment. It is perceived to be a source of fuel for us to carry on and perform our daily tasks optimally. We need the nutrients and minerals that we get from food to make sure that our bodies can function their regular processes properly. We need food to aid in the growth and development of our bones, muscles, and organs.

We need food for the energy to achieve our goals and make our mark on the world.

From a more artistic and emotional perspective, food is seen as a form of expression. Sometimes, one's dietary habits are merely manifestations of a person's feelings or mood at the time. We have always seen how food is often designated as the centerpiece behind a celebration or gathering among people. Food is able to connect and bring people together. Food is a manifestation of culture and heritage. Food is a symbolism of ideas and values. Food can even be a solution for heartaches and disappointments the same way that it can supplement achievement and success.

Regardless of how you choose to perceive food in your life, it's important to pay close attention to what you are eating. You always want to be staying aware of what it is you are putting inside of your mouth. After all, part of what makes life meaningful is the element of structure and having a purpose for the things you do. You should have this same kind of approach when it comes to nutrition as well. If you want to make sure that your food is nourishing you in the right way, then you need to be paying closer attention to its nutritional components. If you want to really enjoy the taste and culinary experience of your food, then you have to try to do so purposefully. If you see food as a tool to make you fitter and healthier, then you have to be staying mindful of what you're eating and how much of it you're consuming.

Whether or not you are a practitioner of the keto diet is irrelevant. It pays to stay mindful of your food. After all, food might quite figuratively be what makes the world go round. It's something that continually binds us as a species. It isn't too far fetched to believe that food should always play a very important role in your life. Your culinary philosophies and gastronomic experiences are your own, and you should definitely up to them. There is nothing to be ashamed about taking ownership of what you eat.

Bibliography

39 Keto Comfort Food Recipes for People Who Love Cozy Meals. (2019, March 14). Retrieved from https://blog.bulletproof.com/comfort-food-recipes-keto-paleo-2b2g3c3g4t/

Afshin, A., Sur, P., Cornaby, L., Fay, K., Ferrera, G., & Salama, J. (2019). Health effects of dietary risks in 195 countries, 1990–2017: A systematic analysis for the Global Burden of Disease Study 2017 [Abstract]. Retrieved from https://www.thelancet.com/article/S0140-6736(19)30041-8/fulltext#.

Allen, B. G., Bhatia, S. K., Anderson, C. M., Eichenberger-Gilmore, J. M., Sibenaller, Z. A., Mapuskar, K. A., . . . Fath, M. A. (2014). Keto-genic diets as an adjuvant cancer therapy: History and potential mechanism. *Redox Biology,2*, 963-970. doi:10.1016/j.redox.2014.08.002

Duncan, E. (2019, January 14). Topic: Diets and Weight Loss in the U.S. Retrieved from https://www.statista.com/topics/4392/diets-and-weight-loss-in-the-us/

Easter, M. (2019, July 17). Inside the Rise of Keto: How an Extreme Diet Went Mainstream. Retrieved from https://www.menshealth.com/nutrition/a25775330/keto-diet-history/

Gotter, A. (2017, August 31). Keto diet: Benefits and nutrients. Retrieved from https://www.medicalnewstoday.com/articles/319196.php

Gunnars, K. (2018, November 20). 10 Health Benefits of Low-Carb and Ketogenic Diets. Retrieved from https://www.healthline.com/nutrition/10-benefits-of-low-carb-ketogenic-diets

Krampf, M. (2018, December 19). 18 Low-Carb Keto Comfort Food Recipes to Get You Through Winter. Retrieved from https://parade.com/

847066/mayakrampf/18-low-carb-keto-com-
fort-food-recipes-to-get-you-through-winter/

Szewczyk, J. (2019, July 11). 16 Hearty Low-Carb
Dinners That Are Totally Keto-Friendly. Retrieved from https://www.buzzfeed.com/
jesseszewczyk/low-carb-keto-comfort-food-re-
cipes

Your Guide to the Pros and Cons of the Keto
Diet. (2019, July 08). Retrieved from https://
ketologic.com/article/the-ketogenic-diet-pros-
and-cons-of-a-low-carb-high-fat-way-of-eating/

Made in the USA
Monee, IL
13 November 2023

46393138R00074